HEMORRHOIDS DISEASE COOKBOOK FOR BEGINNERS

A Natural Home Remedy Approach to Treating and Preventing Hemorrhoid Disease with Over 75 High Fiber, Low Fat Diet Recipes

Sarah Jordan, LD, CCN

COPYRIGHT PAGE

Copyright © 2023 by Sarah Jordan, LD, CCN

The information and recipes in The Ketogenic Diet for Enhancing Cardiovascular Health are not meant to replace professional medical or nutritional advice and are provided solely for educational reasons. The author and publisher disclaim all liability for any harm that may come from following the advice in this book. Before making any modifications to one's diet or beginning a program to lose weight, it is recommended that the reader seek the advice of a healthcare provider or nutritionist.

Table of Contents

CHAPTER I: INTRODUCTION TO THE HEMORRHOIDS DIET

The recipes in this book will take you on a journey of healing and sustenance. In these chapters, you'll learn how to enjoy a delicious and healthy diet while taking care of the pain associated with hemorrhoids. Even though hemorrhoids are rather common, they can still be a bother. Don't fret, though; this cookbook is meant to help you heal and develop a healthy relationship with food.

This cookbook discusses the role of nutrition in the treatment of hemorrhoids. Our goal is to arm you with as much information, advice, and delicious recipes as possible that adhere to the principles of a diet that is safe for those with hemorrhoids. We recognize the difficulties you have in dealing with this disease and are here to help you in any way we can.

The next chapters will introduce you to the concepts of eating fiber-rich meals, staying hydrated, and practicing mindful eating. You'll learn why and how specific meals might help your digestive system feel better. We've put up a compilation of dishes that are both nutritious and delicious. We hope that you enjoy and benefit from your gastronomic adventure with us, from filling breakfasts to delicious meals and healthy snacks.

In this book, you will not only find recipes that are easy on the digestive system, but also procedures for cooking that maintain the food's nutritious worth. In addition to discussing food, we will also discuss how a change in lifestyle might aid in the treatment of hemorrhoids. We're thrilled to be a part of the overall improvement of your health, so please keep that in mind.

Keep in mind that getting expert advice is crucial before starting this enterprise. This cookbook is meant to supplement your existing resources, not replace them, on your path to health and wellness.

We're happy to be a part of your journey, whether it's to try something new, get healthier, or alleviate pain. Dive into the world of hemorrhoid-friendly cooking with me and learn the pleasures of eating for health, one healthy meal at a time.

What are Hemorrhoids?

Hemorrhoids, often known as piles, are a vascular disorder that affects the area below the rectum and the anus. Hemorrhoids are caused by the swelling, inflammation, or distention of the blood vessels that play a critical role in controlling bowel motions. This ailment can range from being somewhat irritating to quite painful and inconvenient.

There are two primary kinds of hemorrhoids: internal and external. Hemorrhoids on the interior of the rectum are not usually obvious to others. They might lead to a sense of fullness or discomfort and even bleeding during bowel movements. On the other hand, external hemorrhoids manifest as painful bumps on the skin just outside of the anus. These external hemorrhoids can be itchy, painful, and uncomfortable, especially when seated or bowel movements are involved.

Hemorrhoids can be caused by a number of things, including being sedentary, being overweight, having constipation, having diarrhea, being pregnant, or having a bowel movement that takes too long. However, factors such as age and genetic predisposition might also contribute to their emergence. Poor eating habits, in particular a lack of dietary fiber, can aggravate hemorrhoids by making feces too hard and painful to pass, which can cause more bleeding.

Hemorrhoids are a frequent health problem, but they may be treated with dietary changes, lifestyle modifications, and even surgical procedures in extreme situations. This cookbook is intended to help you make healthier food choices and gain knowledge into the role nutrition plays in the development and progression of hemorrhoids. Because hemorrhoids can manifest differently in different people, it's necessary to have a professional medical opinion to ensure a proper diagnosis and effective treatment.

Causes and Risk Factors

Many people believe that hemorrhoids develop when the blood vessels in the rectal and anal areas get irritated or stretched. They can affect anyone, but there are more likely to be particular causes and risk factors that contribute to their development.

Constant exertion when defecating is a major contributor. Hemorrhoids are a result of the growth and bulging of blood vessels in the rectal region, which can be caused by chronic straining when trying to evacuate feces. Constipation is a common cause of this stress since it makes defecating more difficult and raises blood pressure throughout the body.

Lack of dietary fiber is another prevalent cause of hemorrhoids. Fiber serves a critical function in adding weight to stools and facilitating regular bowel movements, hence a lack of fiber in the diet can contribute to constipation. Hemorrhoids may form from a diet deficient in fiber since it causes constipation and makes bowel movements more difficult.

Hemorrhoids risk is increased by being overweight. Veins in the lower pelvic area swell and become more prone to irritation when subjected to the additional pressure that comes with being overweight. Hemorrhoids can be caused by poor blood circulation, which is hindered by a sedentary lifestyle that frequently goes hand in hand with obesity.

Hemorrhoids are more likely to occur during pregnancy than at any other time. In addition to hormonal changes, the increased strain on the abdomen and pelvic region that occurs during pregnancy can cause blood vessels to enlarge. Hemorrhoids can also be caused by the strain that many women endure during labor and delivery.

The aging process may also play a role since the tissues that support the anal area's blood arteries might deteriorate over time. Hemorrhoids are more common in the elderly because of this.

Hemorrhoid vulnerability may also be influenced by genetics. Hemorrhoids may run in families because of inherited characteristics that influence the health of blood vessels and the body's inflammatory response.

In conclusion, there is no one cause or risk factor that consistently causes hemorrhoids. Constant straining when passing feces, inadequate fiber intake, obesity, inactivity, pregnancy, advanced age, and genetic susceptibility are all risk factors. Some of these characteristics are modifiable by alterations to one's way of life, while others are innate or can call for more nuanced approaches to treatment. In order to take the necessary precautions and seek the proper medical advice for efficient hemorrhoid treatment, it is crucial to be aware of the reasons and risk factors involved.

Common Symptoms and Discomfort

Although hemorrhoids are rather common, they can cause a wide variety of symptoms and degrees of difficulty in different people. Rectal and anal blood vessel inflammation and edema are at the heart of these symptoms.

Rectal bleeding is a common sign of hemorrhoids. This happens when the irritated and bleeding enlarged internal or exterior blood vessels develop during bowel motions. The blood is usually a vivid shade of red, and it may be easily spotted on toilet paper or in the bowl. Rectal bleeding might be frightening, but it's important to see a doctor to rule out more serious reasons.

An itchy genital area is another annoying symptom. Hemorrhoids can produce discomforting itching due to inflammation and dampness. Itching the region just makes things worse since it irritates the skin even more.

Hemorrhoids, especially those on the outside, are frequently accompanied with pain. When a blood clot develops inside of external hemorrhoids, a condition known as thrombosis, the hemorrhoids become highly sensitive and painful. Sitting, standing, or even walking can be painful due to this discomfort, which is typically characterized as acute and stabbing.

Hemorrhoids often cause pain or difficulty while urinating or defecating. When blood vessels are already inflamed, passing feces, especially those that are firm, might irritate and put pressure on them. This can cause discomfort in the rectal region before and after bowel motions, including a sense of fullness, heaviness, or pain.

External hemorrhoids are characterized by a protrusion or swelling around the anus. It is possible to see and feel lumps or bulges around the anus opening caused by enlarged blood vessels. These growths might aggravate preexisting conditions including pain and itching.

A feeling of incomplete bowel evacuation or a feeling that something is trapped can occur in situations of prolapsed internal hemorrhoids, when they protrude out of the anus. Because of this, you may find yourself straining more than necessary every time you have to go to the bathroom.

Perhaps while these are classic signs of hemorrhoids, they can also point to other medical problems including anal fissures or perhaps something more catastrophic. Therefore, it is essential to obtain a professional diagnosis in order to guarantee effective management and alleviation of discomfort.

In conclusion, the symptoms and sensations associated with hemorrhoids can range from rectal bleeding to itching to pain to difficulty passing stool to the development of bloated or protruding lumps. These symptoms can range from mild to severe, and they can have a significant impact on everyday living if not treated properly.

CHAPTER II: BENEFITS OF EXPLORING A HEMORRHOIDS-FRIENDLY DIET

A diet that is easy on the hemorrhoids may be a powerful tool in the fight against and management of this problem. What we eat has an immediate effect on our digestive health, so being mindful about what we eat may help reduce discomfort and improve our health in general.

Increasing fiber consumption is a cornerstone of a diet designed to alleviate hemorrhoids. High-fiber diets result in softer, more manageable bowel movements. Because of this, you won't have to strain as much when you go to the bathroom, which is a primary cause of hemorrhoids. Hemorrhoids are often brought on by constipation, which may be avoided by eating high-fiber meals such whole grains, fruits, vegetables, and legumes.

Fiber's positive effects extend beyond its role in digestion to include stabilizing blood sugar. Those who are overweight or who suffer from diabetes should pay special attention to this, since stable blood sugar levels might indirectly aid with hemorrhoid control. Foods high in fiber have a lower glycemic index and are digested more slowly, both of which contribute to more consistent blood sugar levels.

Another important part of a diet that helps with hemorrhoids is drinking enough of water. Water consumption helps maintain a soft stool, which is easier to pass through the digestive tract. When you're dehydrated, your stools become more difficult to pass, which might cause you to strain, which can aggravate your hemorrhoids. Water-dense fruits and vegetables, as well as herbal teas, can help you stay properly hydrated.

The best way to alleviate irritation and pain is to eat meals that are easy on the digestive system. Hemorrhoid symptoms, such as itching and irritation, can be made worse by consuming spicy foods, coffee, or alcohol. In order to get the nutrients you need while reducing your exposure to allergens, try eating more whole, unprocessed foods, lean proteins, and healthy fats.

One further benefit of a hemorrhoid-friendly diet is improved weight control. Hemorrhoids are more likely to occur in people who are overweight, since the extra weight puts strain on the veins and arteries in the anal region. Supporting hemorrhoid control, a diet high in nutrient-dense, low-calorie meals can aid in achieving and maintaining a healthy weight.

In the end, a diet that helps with hemorrhoids does more than just alleviate symptoms; it gives people the tools they need to take responsibility of their digestive health and overall wellness. Reduce the pain and irritation caused by hemorrhoids and increase your sensation of control and vigor by eating more fiber-rich foods, drinking enough of water, and making more conscious dietary choices. However, keep in mind that the key to successfully treating this ailment is a multifaceted strategy that may include medical supervision and changes to one's way of life.

Incorporating Fiber-Rich Foods and their benefits

Hemorrhoid management and improved digestive health both begin with a diet that includes plenty of foods high in fiber. The tension that might increase hemorrhoid symptoms can be alleviated with the help of fiber, which plays a critical role in promoting smooth and regular bowel movements. Including a wide range of high-fiber foods in your daily diet can have various positive effects on your health.

If you want to start eating more fiber, whole grains are a great place to start. Insoluble fiber, found in foods like whole wheat bread, brown rice, quinoa, and oats, makes stools bulkier and easier to pass through the digestive tract. These grains are great for avoiding the pain and irritation of hemorrhoids, and they also assist with constipation.

Pulses and legumes like beans, lentils, and chickpeas are also excellent sources of fiber. They are an excellent source of both fiber and plant-based protein. Including these items in your diet will help you feel full and promote good digestion. Indirectly aiding with hemorrhoid treatment, the soluble fiber included in legumes can help keep blood sugar levels stable.

Fruits and vegetables of various hues are crucial to a balanced, fiber-rich diet. Constipation can be avoided because to the soluble and insoluble fiber included in them. You can't go wrong with anything from broccoli to apples. The digestive and immunological systems both benefit from a wide range of nutrients found in fruits and vegetables of different hues.

Both flaxseeds and chia seeds are incredibly nutritious and a great source of fiber. These small seeds have a high concentration of soluble fiber, which turns into a gel when mixed with water. Stools can be made easier to transit through the digestive tract by doing this. Smoothies, yogurt, and oatmeal can all benefit from a sprinkling of these seeds to increase their fiber content.

You may avoid constipation, relieve the pain of hemorrhoids, and encourage a thriving gut microbiota by eating more of these fiber-rich foods. Feeding the good bacteria in the digestive tract and intestines has been linked to improved digestion, immunity, and general health.

To minimize gastrointestinal distress, remember to gradually increase your fiber intake. Along with eating fiber-rich meals, it's crucial to drink enough of water to assist the fiber do its work. By including these nutritious items into your diet, you'll not only reduce your hemorrhoid symptoms, but also improve your digestive health and feel better overall.

Foods to Avoid: Triggers and Irritants

Hemorrhoid management and the avoidance of discomfort are greatly aided by avoiding foods that might function as triggers or irritants. You may prevent the worsening of hemorrhoid symptoms and improve your digestive health by simply avoiding the foods listed above from your diet.

Hemorrhoid sufferers are warned to avoid spicy meals at all costs. Capsaicin-rich spices, in particular, can aggravate anal inflammation and irritate the gastrointestinal system.

Because of the potential for increased itching, burning, and discomfort after eating spicy foods, it is best to limit or avoid them.

Foods containing caffeine and alcohol are also on the watch list. Both drugs can cause you to lose water, which can make your stools tougher and make it more difficult to pass them. Hemorrhoid pain and healing time can both be slowed by a lack of fluids. To stay hydrated, it's best to avoid or consume caffeinated beverages (including coffee and some types of tea) and alcoholic beverages in moderation.

Constipation and other digestive problems have been linked to a diet heavy in processed foods that are also high in refined sugars and harmful fats. These meals are low in fiber and other nutrients essential for proper digestion, which may make bowel movements more difficult and uncomfortable. Hemorrhoid sufferers would do well to limit their consumption of sugary snacks, deep-fried meals, and highly processed snacks, or to swap them out for healthier options.

Some people have reactions to dairy products, especially those with a high fat content. Constipation and other bowel movement problems may be exacerbated by dairy consumption. If you have IBS and find that dairy products make your symptoms worse, switching to low-fat or dairy-free options may help.

Consuming an excessive amount of red meat, such a roast, can be difficult for the digestive system and may even cause constipation. Reduce your consumption and switch to leaner cuts instead of eliminating it altogether. Plant-based protein sources are great for your digestive health and can help you keep your diet in check.

Hemorrhoid pain can be made worse by eating processed meals like fast food and packaged snacks, which are poor in fiber and heavy in salt. These foods often aren't very nourishing and might actually make you feel worse.

You may help your efforts to control hemorrhoids by eating better by being aware of these possible triggers and irritants. It's not essential to cut out these meals entirely, but knowledge and moderation are crucial. It's important to pay attention to how different meals affect your body because everyone has a unique physiology. This will help you figure out what you need to avoid or take in moderation to feel your best.

CHAPTER III: PRESERVING NUTRIENTS THE HEALTHY WAY

It's not just what you eat, but also how you eat, that matters when you're on a diet for hemorrhoids. By choosing healthful cooking techniques, you may keep more of the nutrients in your food while also making it easier on your digestive system.

Steaming is a low-heat cooking method that allows food's natural flavors and nutrients to shine through. Steaming veggies rather than boiling them preserves the water-soluble vitamins and minerals. Vegetables are more easily digested after being steamed, and their brilliant colors and tastes are preserved in the process.

Another versatile and healthy cooking method is roasting, which can be used for a wide range of foods. The natural sugars and tastes of vegetables and lean meats may be brought out and enhanced by roasting them with a sprinkle of healthy oil. The natural sugars in the food are caramelized, giving it a delicious flavor while the vital nutrients are kept intact.

If you want to give your dish a smokey taste without using a lot of oil or fat, grilling is a terrific alternative. When grilling, choose marinades that are both tasty and gentle on your digestive tract if you suffer from hemorrhoids. Grilled foods are a great way to spice up your diet and try something new.

Vegetables and lean meats may be prepared rapidly and healthfully in a stir-fry. Foods may be cooked quickly while still maintaining their color, texture, and nutritional value by using a tiny quantity of healthy oil in a hot pan. As an added bonus, stir-frying is a great way to get in a rainbow of healthy veggies.

Foods with harder fibers can be made more digestible by slow cooking, which is also a time-efficient way. Beans and other legumes, which are high in fiber and plant-based proteins, benefit greatly from this technique. In addition to producing tasty and delicate food, the slow and low cooking method also helps preserve the nutritional worth of the components.

Certain foods can be cooked well by boiling, but it is crucial to incorporate the cooking liquid into the dish so that no nutrients are lost. Soups and broths made from vegetables or lean meats boiled in water, for instance, have a nourishing basis that might be good for hydration and digestive comfort.

Hemorrhoid sufferers should be careful while cooking with fatty ingredients, strong spices, and other irritants since they might make the condition worse. To add taste without pain, try utilizing herbs, spices, and seasonings that grow naturally.

You may make tasty and nutrient-rich meals that are helpful for your hemorrhoids diet by choosing these healthy cooking methods and focusing on fresh, whole ingredients. Eating meals that are mild on your digestive system and simple to digest will help you feel better overall and give you more energy.

Fluid Intake and Hydration

Hemorrhoid treatment and intestinal wellness benefit greatly from enough fluid consumption. Constipation is a major cause of hemorrhoid pain, and drinking enough water can help ease the symptoms and avoid them altogether.

Keeping stools soft and simple to pass by drinking water often throughout the day. To avoid irritating and inflaming the blood vessels in the anal region, it is important to have soft stools that limit the need to strain during bowel movements. Hemorrhoid pain can be exacerbated by the strain of passing firm stools, which puts more pressure on the underlying blood vessels.

Drinking herbal teas like chamomile, peppermint, or ginger tea will help you stay hydrated and may help settle your stomach. Without any extra sweeteners or allergens, these teas may provide soothing hydration and aid in smooth digestion.

Water-rich fruits and vegetables are great for keeping you hydrated and your digestive system healthy. Cucumbers, watermelons, oranges, and celery are all examples of water-rich foods that are also good for you since they include vitamins, minerals, and fiber in addition to the water they contain.

Caffeine and alcohol both have diuretic effects, so be aware that drinking too much of either might cause dehydration. Therefore, moderation and equilibrium are essential whether you prefer to drink coffee, tea, soda, beer, wine, or spirits. In order to prevent dehydration, you should drink more water.

Keep in mind that people have different hydration needs according on their age, activity level, environment, and general health. Aim for 8 glasses (64 ounces) of water each day as a general rule of thumb, but pay attention to your body and make any necessary adjustments to your fluid consumption.

Keeping yourself well hydrated can help prevent hemorrhoids from forming or deteriorating in the first place by preserving the health of your tissues and blood vessels. You may help your digestive system, lessen the likelihood of constipation, and improve your comfort and well-being by drinking plenty of water, drinking herbal teas, and eating foods high in water content.

Tailoring the Diet to Individual Needs

Managing hemorrhoids successfully often comes down to making dietary changes that are specific to the person experiencing them. A person's medical history, food preferences, way of life, and current health issues are just a few of the variables that go into establishing the best diet for hemorrhoid treatment.

One of the first things to do when creating a personalized diet is to take into account any food allergies or intolerances the individual may have. Hemorrhoid sufferers should eat a diet that is safe, nutritious, and takes into account any food allergies or intolerances they may have.

In order to tailor the diet to the individual, it is crucial to assess the severity of the hemorrhoid symptoms. While some people may only feel minor pain, those with more severe symptoms may need to make more drastic changes to their diet. It may be especially important for those with severe symptoms to avoid triggers and focus on foods that are easy on the system.

Personal tastes and cultural norms about food intake should also be taken into account. Making the switch to a diet that is better for your hemorrhoids easier by including some of your favorite foods and flavors. Compliance and sustained success are more likely with this strategy.

Dietary adjustments must take into account the individual's medical history and any preexisting illnesses. Hemorrhoid sufferers who simultaneously struggle with diseases like diabetes, heart disease, or gastrointestinal issues require a diet that does more than just treat their symptoms. In such a situation, it is best to seek the advice of a doctor or a trained dietician.

Dietary decisions ought to be influenced by degree of physical activity. It's possible that athletes need more overall calories and certain nutrients to power their exercises and aid in recuperation. The hemorrhoids-friendly diet strikes a balance between these requirements, allowing for optimal digestion and exercise.

It's also important to think about things like your job schedule and social obligations. Adherence to the hemorrhoids-friendly diet can be boosted by making meal planning an integral part of everyday life. Similarly, if you're having trouble sticking to your diet in social situations, finding alternatives to frequent irritants and triggers will assist.

Finally, regular checks and tweaks are essential. It's crucial to monitor how one's body reacts to dietary changes. Modifications can be made if it turns out that a certain diet or eating habit is exacerbating symptoms or slowing recovery.

A person's medical history, symptoms, preferences, and way of life must all be taken into account while developing a hemorrhoids diet plan specifically for that person. This individualized strategy makes dietary changes that help with hemorrhoids last and are in line with broader health objectives. A licensed dietician or healthcare provider can help you develop a nutrition plan that is tailored to your specific needs and goals, allowing you to feel your best.

CHAPTER IV: HEMORRHOIDS FRIENDLY RECIPES

HEMORRHOIDS FRIENDLY BREAKFAST RECIPES

Plain Oatmeal with Sliced Bananas:

Ingredients

1/2 cup rolled oats

1 cup water or milk (dairy or plant-based)

Pinch of salt

1 banana, sliced

Instructions

In a saucepan, bring the water or milk to a boil.

Add the rolled oats and a pinch of salt, then reduce the heat to a simmer.

Cook the oats, stirring occasionally, for about 5 minutes or until they reach your desired consistency.

Remove from heat and transfer the oatmeal to a bowl.

Top with sliced bananas and enjoy.

Greek Yogurt with Mixed Berries:

Ingredients

1 cup Greek yogurt

1/2 cup mixed berries (such as blueberries, strawberries, raspberries)

Instructions

Spoon the Greek yogurt into a bowl.

Wash and prepare the mixed berries.

Top the yogurt with the mixed berries and enjoy.

Scrambled Eggs with Sautéed Spinach:

Ingredients

2 large eggs

1 cup fresh spinach leaves

Salt and pepper to taste

Olive oil or cooking spray

Instructions

Heat a non-stick skillet over medium heat and add a little olive oil or cooking spray.

Add the fresh spinach leaves and sauté until wilted, about 1-2 minutes.

In a bowl, whisk the eggs and season with salt and pepper.

Pour the whisked eggs into the skillet with the sautéed spinach.

Cook, stirring gently, until the eggs are scrambled and fully cooked.

Transfer to a plate and serve.

Whole Grain Toast with Avocado Spread:

Ingredients

2 slices whole grain bread, toasted

1 ripe avocado

Salt and pepper to taste

Optional toppings: red pepper flakes, sliced radishes

Instructions

Cut the ripe avocado in half, remove the pit, and scoop out the flesh into a bowl.

Mash the avocado with a fork until smooth.

Spread the mashed avocado onto the toasted whole grain bread slices.

Sprinkle with salt and pepper, and add optional toppings if desired.

Serve the avocado toast.

Fresh Fruit Salad with a Drizzle of Honey:

Ingredients

Assorted fresh fruits (such as melon, grapes, kiwi, oranges, etc.)

Honey for drizzling

Instructions

Wash, peel, and cut the fresh fruits into bite-sized pieces.

Combine the assorted fruits in a bowl.

Drizzle a small amount of honey over the fruit salad.

Gently toss the fruit salad to combine.

Serve the fruit salad in bowls.

Cottage Cheese with Sliced Peaches:

Ingredients

1 cup low-fat cottage cheese

1 ripe peach, sliced

Instructions

Spoon the cottage cheese into a bowl.

Wash, pit, and slice the ripe peach.

Arrange the sliced peaches over the cottage cheese.

Enjoy the cottage cheese and peach combination.

Poached Eggs with Whole Wheat English Muffin:

Ingredients

2 eggs

1 whole wheat English muffin, toasted

Vinegar (for poaching)

Salt and pepper to taste

Instructions

Fill a deep skillet with water and add a splash of vinegar.

Heat the water until it's simmering, not boiling.

Crack each egg into a small cup.

Gently slide the eggs into the simmering water one by one.

Poach the eggs for about 3-4 minutes until the whites are set but the yolks are still runny.

Use a slotted spoon to carefully remove the poached eggs from the water.

Place the poached eggs on toasted whole wheat English muffins.

Season with salt and pepper.

Serve the poached eggs on the English muffins.

Smoothie with Kale, Pineapple, and Almond Milk:

Ingredients

1 cup kale leaves, stems removed

1 cup frozen pineapple chunks

1 cup almond milk (or any milk of your choice)

Optional: honey or agave syrup for sweetness

Instructions

Wash the kale leaves thoroughly.

In a blender, combine the kale, frozen pineapple chunks, and almond milk.

Blend until smooth and creamy.

Taste and add honey or agave syrup if desired for extra sweetness.

Pour the smoothie into a glass and enjoy.

Low-Fat Yogurt Parfait with Granola and Kiwi:

Ingredients

1 cup low-fat yogurt (plain or flavored)

1/4 cup granola

1 kiwi, peeled and diced

Instructions

In a glass or bowl, layer the low-fat yogurt.

Add a layer of diced kiwi on top of the yogurt.

Sprinkle a layer of granola over the kiwi.

Repeat the layers if desired.

Serve the parfait with a spoon.

Breakfast Quinoa with Diced Apples and Cinnamon:

Ingredients

1/2 cup quinoa

1 cup water or milk (dairy or plant-based)

1 apple, diced

1/2 teaspoon cinnamon

Optional: chopped nuts or seeds for topping

Instructions

Rinse the quinoa thoroughly under cold water.

In a saucepan, combine quinoa and water or milk. Bring to a boil.

Reduce heat to a simmer, cover, and cook for about 15 minutes or until the liquid is absorbed and quinoa is tender.

Fluff the quinoa with a fork and let it cool slightly.

Stir in the diced apple and cinnamon.

Top with chopped nuts or seeds if desired.

Serve the breakfast quinoa warm.

Whole Grain Cereal with Almond Milk and Strawberries:

Ingredients

1 cup whole grain cereal (such as muesli or bran flakes)

1 cup almond milk (or any milk of your choice)

Fresh strawberries, sliced

Instructions

Place the whole grain cereal in a bowl.

Pour almond milk over the cereal.

Add sliced strawberries on top.

Let the cereal soak in the almond milk for a few minutes before eating.

Enjoy the cereal with strawberries and almond milk.

Veggie Omelette with Bell Peppers and Onions:

Ingredients

2 large eggs

1/4 cup diced bell peppers (any color)

1/4 cup diced onions

Salt and pepper to taste

Olive oil or cooking spray

Instructions

Heat a non-stick skillet over medium heat and add a little olive oil or cooking spray.

Add the diced bell peppers and onions. Sauté for a few minutes until they soften.

In a bowl, whisk the eggs and season with salt and pepper.

Pour the whisked eggs into the skillet over the sautéed veggies.

Cook until the edges set, then gently lift the edges with a spatula to let uncooked egg flow underneath.

Once the omelette is mostly set but still slightly runny on top, fold it in half.

Cook for another minute or until fully cooked.

Slide the omelette onto a plate and serve.

Rice Cake Topped with Almond Butter and Sliced Pears:

Ingredients

1 rice cake

2 tablespoons almond butter

1 pear, thinly sliced

Instructions

Spread almond butter onto the rice cake.

Arrange the sliced pears on top of the almond butter.

Enjoy the rice cake with almond butter and sliced pears.

Steamed Sweet Potatoes with a Sprinkle of Cinnamon:

Ingredients

1 small sweet potato

Ground cinnamon

Instructions

Wash the sweet potato and peel if desired.

Cut the sweet potato into bite-sized pieces.

Steam the sweet potato until tender, about 10-15 minutes.

Place the steamed sweet potato in a bowl.

Sprinkle ground cinnamon over the sweet potato.

Toss gently to coat with cinnamon.

Serve the steamed sweet potatoes with a hint of cinnamon.

Whole Wheat Waffles with a Side of Mixed Fruit:

Ingredients

2 whole wheat waffles (store-bought or homemade)

Assorted mixed fruit (such as berries, sliced bananas, kiwi, etc.)

Instructions

Toast the whole wheat waffles according to package instructions or your preference.

Arrange the toasted waffles on a plate.

Wash, peel, and prepare the mixed fruit.

Serve the waffles with a side of mixed fruit.

HEMORRHOIDS FRIENDLY LUNCH RECIPES

Grilled Chicken Salad with Mixed Greens:

Ingredients

1 grilled chicken breast, sliced

Mixed greens (lettuce, spinach, arugula, etc.)

Cherry tomatoes, halved

Cucumber, sliced

Red onion, thinly sliced

Balsamic vinaigrette dressing

Instructions

Arrange the mixed greens on a plate.

Add the sliced grilled chicken, cherry tomatoes, cucumber, and red onion.

Drizzle with balsamic vinaigrette dressing.

Toss the salad gently and enjoy.

Quinoa and Black Bean Bowl with Salsa:

Ingredients

1 cup cooked quinoa

1 cup black beans, drained and rinsed

Salsa (store-bought or homemade)

Fresh cilantro, chopped

Lime wedges

Instructions

In a bowl, combine cooked quinoa and black beans.

Top with salsa and chopped cilantro.

Squeeze lime juice over the bowl.

Mix well and enjoy.

Vegetable Stir-Fry with Tofu and Brown Rice:

Ingredients

1 cup firm tofu, cubed

Assorted vegetables (bell peppers, broccoli, carrots, snap peas, etc.)

Low-sodium soy sauce

Sesame oil

Cooked brown rice

Instructions

Heat a skillet or wok with a little sesame oil.

Add cubed tofu and stir-fry until lightly browned.

Add assorted vegetables and stir-fry until they're tender-crisp.

Drizzle with low-sodium soy sauce and toss.

Serve the stir-fried vegetables and tofu over cooked brown rice.

Turkey and Avocado Wrap in a Whole Wheat Tortilla:

Ingredients

1 whole wheat tortilla

Sliced turkey breast

Avocado, sliced

Lettuce leaves

Tomato, sliced

Mustard or mayonnaise (optional)

Instructions

Lay the whole wheat tortilla flat.

Place slices of turkey, avocado, lettuce, and tomato on the tortilla.

Add a drizzle of mustard or mayonnaise if desired.

Roll up the tortilla, folding in the sides as you go.

Slice in half and enjoy the wrap.

Baked Salmon with Steamed Vegetables:

Ingredients

1 salmon fillet

Lemon juice

Olive oil

Assorted vegetables (broccoli, carrots, zucchini, etc.)

Instructions

Preheat the oven and line a baking sheet with parchment paper.

Place the salmon fillet on the baking sheet.

Drizzle with lemon juice and olive oil.

Bake until the salmon is cooked through.

Steam the assorted vegetables until tender.

Serve the baked salmon with steamed vegetables.

Hummus and Vegetable Wrap:

Ingredients

1 whole wheat tortilla

Hummus

Assorted vegetables (bell peppers, cucumbers, carrots, etc.)

Baby spinach leaves

Instructions

Spread a layer of hummus onto the whole wheat tortilla.

Add sliced vegetables and baby spinach on top of the hummus.

Roll up the tortilla, folding in the sides as you go.

Slice in half and enjoy the wrap.

Greek Yogurt and Cucumber Tzatziki with Pita Bread:

Ingredients

1 cup Greek yogurt

Cucumber, grated and squeezed to remove excess moisture

Garlic, minced

Fresh dill, chopped

Lemon juice

Whole wheat pita bread

Instructions

In a bowl, combine Greek yogurt, grated cucumber, minced garlic, chopped dill, and lemon juice.

Mix well to make the tzatziki sauce.

Warm the whole wheat pita bread.

Serve the Greek yogurt tzatziki with pita bread for dipping or spreading.

Chickpea and Vegetable Curry with Basmati Rice:

Ingredients

1 cup cooked chickpeas (canned or cooked from dry)

Assorted vegetables (bell peppers, carrots, peas, etc.)

Curry powder or paste

Coconut milk

Cooked basmati rice

Instructions

In a skillet, sauté assorted vegetables until slightly tender.

Add cooked chickpeas and a spoonful of curry powder or paste.

Pour in coconut milk and let it simmer until flavors combine.

Serve the chickpea curry over cooked basmati rice.

Caprese Salad with Fresh Mozzarella, Tomatoes, and Basil:

Ingredients

Fresh mozzarella cheese, sliced

Tomatoes, sliced

Fresh basil leaves

Balsamic glaze or vinegar

Olive oil

Salt and pepper to taste

Instructions

Arrange slices of fresh mozzarella and tomatoes on a plate.

Tuck fresh basil leaves between the cheese and tomatoes.

Drizzle with balsamic glaze or vinegar and olive oil.

Season with salt and pepper.

Enjoy the simple Caprese salad.

Grilled Vegetable and Feta Cheese Quinoa Bowl:

Ingredients

Assorted vegetables (zucchini, eggplant, bell peppers, etc.)

Olive oil

Cooked quinoa

Feta cheese, crumbled

Lemon zest

Fresh parsley, chopped

Instructions

Toss assorted vegetables with olive oil and grill until tender.

Arrange grilled vegetables over cooked quinoa.

Sprinkle with crumbled feta cheese, lemon zest, and chopped parsley.

Serve the grilled vegetable and feta cheese quinoa bowl.

Whole Grain Pasta with Marinara Sauce and Sautéed Spinach:

Ingredients

Whole grain pasta

Marinara sauce (store-bought or homemade)

Fresh spinach leaves

Olive oil

Garlic, minced

Red pepper flakes (optional)

Instructions

Cook whole grain pasta according to package instructions.

In a skillet, heat olive oil and sauté minced garlic and red pepper flakes.

Add fresh spinach and cook until wilted.

Toss cooked pasta with marinara sauce and sautéed spinach.

Serve the whole grain pasta with marinara and spinach.

Tuna Salad with Mixed Greens and Olive Oil Dressing:

Ingredients

Canned tuna, drained

Mixed greens

Cherry tomatoes, halved

Red onion, thinly sliced

Olive oil

Lemon juice

Dijon mustard

Salt and pepper to taste

Instructions

In a bowl, combine canned tuna, mixed greens, cherry tomatoes, and red onion.

In a separate bowl, whisk together olive oil, lemon juice, Dijon mustard, salt, and pepper to make the dressing.

Drizzle the dressing over the salad and toss to coat.

Enjoy the tuna salad with mixed greens.

Roast Beef and Vegetable Wrap:

Ingredients

1 whole wheat tortilla

Sliced roast beef

Sliced cheese (optional)

Assorted vegetables (lettuce, tomato, cucumber, etc.)

Mustard or horseradish sauce (optional)

Instructions

Lay the whole wheat tortilla flat.

Place slices of roast beef and cheese (if using) on the tortilla.

Add sliced vegetables and a drizzle of mustard or horseradish sauce if desired.

Roll up the tortilla, folding in the sides as you go.

Slice in half and enjoy the wrap.

Spinach and Mushroom Omelette:

Ingredients

3 eggs

Fresh spinach leaves

Sliced mushrooms

Shredded cheese (such as cheddar or feta)

Salt and pepper to taste

Olive oil or butter

Instructions

In a bowl, beat the eggs and season with salt and pepper.

Heat a non-stick skillet with a little olive oil or butter.

Add sliced mushrooms and sauté until they release moisture.

Add fresh spinach leaves and cook until wilted.

Pour the beaten eggs over the vegetables.

Sprinkle shredded cheese on one half of the omelette.

Once the eggs are set, fold the omelette in half.

Cook for another minute until the cheese melts.

Slide the omelette onto a plate and serve.

Sweet Potato and Black Bean Burrito:

Ingredients

1 large sweet potato, roasted and mashed

1 cup cooked black beans

Whole wheat tortilla

Salsa or pico de gallo

Avocado, sliced

Fresh cilantro, chopped

Instructions

Lay the whole wheat tortilla flat.

Spread mashed sweet potato over the tortilla.

Add cooked black beans, salsa or pico de gallo, avocado slices, and chopped cilantro.

Roll up the tortilla, folding in the sides as you go.

Slice in half and enjoy the sweet potato and black bean burrito.

HEMORRHOIDS FRIENDLY DINNER RECIPES

Grilled Chicken Breast with Roasted Vegetables:

Ingredients

1 boneless, skinless chicken breast

Assorted vegetables (bell peppers, zucchini, carrots, etc.)

Olive oil

Herbs and spices (such as rosemary, thyme, garlic powder)

Salt and pepper to taste

Instructions

Preheat the grill or oven to medium-high heat.

Season the chicken breast with herbs, spices, salt, and pepper.

Grill or bake the chicken until cooked through, about 6-8 minutes per side (internal temperature of 165°F or 74°C).

Toss assorted vegetables with olive oil, salt, and pepper.

Roast the vegetables in the oven until tender.

Serve the grilled chicken with roasted vegetables.

Baked Fish with Steamed Broccoli:

Ingredients

1 fish fillet (salmon, cod, etc.)

Lemon juice

Olive oil

Salt and pepper to taste

Broccoli florets

Instructions

Preheat the oven to 375°F (190°C).

Place the fish fillet on a baking sheet.

Drizzle with lemon juice and olive oil, then season with salt and pepper.

Bake until the fish flakes easily with a fork, about 12-15 minutes.

Steam broccoli florets until tender.

Serve the baked fish with steamed broccoli.

Turkey Meatballs with Whole Wheat Pasta and Tomato Sauce:

Ingredients

Ground turkey

Whole wheat pasta

Tomato sauce (store-bought or homemade)

Fresh herbs (such as basil or parsley), chopped

Garlic, minced

Olive oil

Salt and pepper to taste

Instructions

Preheat the oven to 375°F (190°C).

Mix ground turkey with chopped herbs, minced garlic, salt, and pepper.

Form the mixture into meatballs and place on a baking sheet.

Bake until cooked through, about 15-20 minutes.

Cook whole wheat pasta according to package instructions.

Heat tomato sauce and serve it over cooked pasta with turkey meatballs.

Stir-Fried Tofu with Mixed Vegetables and Brown Rice:

Ingredients

Firm tofu, cubed

Assorted vegetables (bell peppers, snap peas, carrots, etc.)

Low-sodium soy sauce

Sesame oil

Cooked brown rice

Instructions

Heat a skillet or wok with a little sesame oil.

Add cubed tofu and stir-fry until lightly browned.

Add assorted vegetables and stir-fry until they're tender-crisp.

Drizzle with low-sodium soy sauce and toss.

Serve the stir-fried tofu and vegetables over cooked brown rice.

Vegetable and Quinoa Stuffed Bell Peppers:

Ingredients

Bell peppers

Quinoa

Assorted vegetables (zucchini, onion, corn, etc.)

Herbs and spices (such as oregano, cumin, paprika)

Olive oil

Shredded cheese (optional)

Instructions

Preheat the oven to 375°F (190°C).

Cut the tops off bell peppers and remove seeds.

Cook quinoa according to package instructions.

Sauté assorted vegetables with olive oil and herbs.

Mix cooked quinoa with sautéed vegetables.

Stuff the quinoa and vegetable mixture into bell peppers.

Bake until peppers are tender, about 20-25 minutes.

Top with shredded cheese if desired and bake until melted.

Roast Beef with Baked Sweet Potatoes:

Ingredients

Roast beef slices

Sweet potatoes

Olive oil

Herbs (such as rosemary, thyme, or cinnamon)

Salt and pepper to taste

Instructions

Preheat the oven to 400°F (200°C).

Wash and scrub sweet potatoes.

Prick sweet potatoes with a fork and rub with olive oil, herbs, salt, and pepper.

Bake sweet potatoes until tender, about 45-60 minutes.

Warm roast beef slices.

Serve the roast beef with baked sweet potatoes.

Spinach and Mushroom Frittata:

Ingredients

Eggs

Fresh spinach leaves

Sliced mushrooms

Onion, finely chopped

Cheese (such as feta or cheddar), crumbled or grated

Salt and pepper to taste

Olive oil or butter

Instructions

Preheat the oven to 375°F (190°C).

In a skillet, sauté chopped onion and sliced mushrooms until softened.

Add fresh spinach leaves and cook until wilted.

Beat eggs in a bowl, season with salt and pepper.

Pour beaten eggs into the skillet over vegetables.

Sprinkle crumbled or grated cheese on top.

Cook on the stovetop for a few minutes until the edges set.

Transfer the skillet to the oven and bake until the frittata is cooked through, about 15-20 minutes.

Slice and serve the spinach and mushroom frittata.

Baked Salmon with Asparagus and Lemon:

Ingredients

Salmon fillet

Lemon slices

Olive oil

Fresh dill (or other herbs)

Salt and pepper to taste

Asparagus spears

Instructions

Preheat the oven to 375°F (190°C).

Place the salmon fillet on a baking sheet.

Drizzle with olive oil, and season with fresh dill, salt, and pepper.

Lay lemon slices on top of the salmon.

Arrange asparagus spears around the salmon.

Bake until the salmon flakes easily with a fork and the asparagus is tender, about 12-15 minutes.

Serve the baked salmon with asparagus and lemon.

Chickpea and Spinach Curry with Basmati Rice:

Ingredients

1 can of chickpeas, drained and rinsed

Fresh spinach leaves

Onion, chopped

Garlic, minced

Curry powder or paste

Coconut milk

Basmati rice

Instructions

Sauté chopped onion and minced garlic until softened.

Add curry powder or paste and cook until fragrant.

Add chickpeas and fresh spinach, stirring until spinach wilts.

Pour in coconut milk and simmer for a few minutes.

Serve the chickpea and spinach curry over cooked basmati rice.

Zucchini Noodles with Marinara Sauce and Grilled Shrimp:

Ingredients

Zucchini, spiralized into noodles

Marinara sauce (store-bought or homemade)

Grilled shrimp

Fresh basil leaves, chopped

Olive oil

Garlic, minced

Instructions

Heat olive oil in a skillet and sauté minced garlic until fragrant.

Add zucchini noodles and sauté for a few minutes until tender.

Warm marinara sauce in a separate pot.

Grill or cook shrimp until cooked through.

Serve zucchini noodles topped with marinara sauce and grilled shrimp.

Garnish with chopped fresh basil.

Grilled Vegetable and Hummus Wrap:

Ingredients

Whole wheat tortilla

Hummus

Grilled assorted vegetables (zucchini, eggplant, bell peppers, etc.)

Baby spinach leaves

Optional: crumbled feta cheese

Instructions

Lay the whole wheat tortilla flat.

Spread a layer of hummus onto the tortilla.

Add grilled vegetables and baby spinach on top of the hummus.

Optionally, sprinkle crumbled feta cheese.

Roll up the tortilla, folding in the sides as you go.

Slice in half and enjoy the wrap.

Quinoa and Black Bean Salad with Lime Vinaigrette:

Ingredients

Cooked quinoa

Black beans, drained and rinsed

Assorted chopped vegetables (tomatoes, bell peppers, red onion, etc.)

Fresh cilantro, chopped

Lime juice

Olive oil

Salt and pepper to taste

Instructions

In a bowl, combine cooked quinoa, black beans, chopped vegetables, and cilantro.

In a separate bowl, whisk together lime juice, olive oil, salt, and pepper to make the vinaigrette.

Drizzle the vinaigrette over the salad and toss to combine.

Serve the quinoa and black bean salad.

Mushroom and Barley Risotto:

Ingredients

Barley

Mushrooms, sliced

Onion, chopped

Vegetable broth

White wine (optional)

Fresh thyme leaves

Parmesan cheese, grated (optional)

Olive oil

Instructions

Sauté chopped onion and sliced mushrooms until mushrooms are browned.

Add barley and stir to coat with oil.

If using, pour in white wine and let it cook off.

Gradually add vegetable broth and cook the barley, stirring frequently.

Stir in fresh thyme leaves and grated Parmesan cheese if desired.

Serve the mushroom and barley risotto.

Roasted Chicken Thighs with Mashed Cauliflower:

Ingredients

Chicken thighs

Olive oil

Herbs (such as rosemary, thyme, or paprika)

Salt and pepper to taste

Cauliflower, chopped

Garlic, minced

Chicken or vegetable broth

Instructions

Preheat the oven to 400°F (200°C).

Rub chicken thighs with olive oil, herbs, salt, and pepper.

Roast the chicken thighs until cooked through, about 30-35 minutes.

Steam or boil cauliflower until tender.

Mash the cooked cauliflower with minced garlic and a splash of chicken or vegetable broth.

Serve the roasted chicken thighs with mashed cauliflower.

Eggplant Parmesan with a Side Salad:

Ingredients

Eggplant, sliced

Bread crumbs

Marinara sauce

Mozzarella cheese, grated

Parmesan cheese, grated

Mixed greens for side salad

Balsamic vinaigrette dressing

Instructions

Preheat the oven to 375°F (190°C).

Dredge eggplant slices in bread crumbs and bake until golden and crispy.

Layer eggplant slices with marinara sauce, mozzarella cheese, and Parmesan cheese.

Bake until cheese is melted and bubbly.

Toss mixed greens with balsamic vinaigrette for the side salad.

Serve the eggplant Parmesan with a side salad.

HEMORRHOIDS FRIENDLY SOUP RECIPES

Minestrone Soup with Whole Wheat Bread:

Ingredients

Assorted vegetables (carrots, celery, zucchini, etc.), diced

Canned diced tomatoes

Cooked kidney beans

Low-sodium vegetable broth

Whole wheat pasta

Herbs and spices (such as oregano, thyme, basil)

Salt and pepper to taste

Instructions

In a pot, sauté diced vegetables in a little olive oil until slightly softened.

Add canned diced tomatoes, cooked kidney beans, and vegetable broth.

Season with herbs, spices, salt, and pepper.

Add whole wheat pasta and simmer until pasta is cooked.

Serve the Minestrone soup with a side of whole wheat bread.

Creamy Tomato Soup with a Side of Mixed Greens:

Ingredients

Canned tomato soup (low-sodium)

Milk or cream (dairy or plant-based)

Herbs (such as basil or thyme)

Mixed greens for side salad

Balsamic vinaigrette dressing

Instructions

Heat canned tomato soup in a pot.

Stir in milk or cream to achieve desired creaminess.

Season with herbs and warm the soup through.

Toss mixed greens with balsamic vinaigrette for the side salad.

Serve the creamy tomato soup with a side of mixed greens.

Chicken and Vegetable Soup with Brown Rice:

Ingredients

Cooked chicken (leftover roasted or poached), shredded

Assorted vegetables (carrots, celery, onion, etc.), diced

Low-sodium chicken broth

Cooked brown rice

Herbs (such as parsley or thyme)

Salt and pepper to taste

Instructions

In a pot, sauté diced vegetables until slightly softened.

Add shredded cooked chicken and chicken broth.

Season with herbs, salt, and pepper.

Simmer until the flavors meld.

Stir in cooked brown rice.

Serve the chicken and vegetable soup.

Spinach and White Bean Soup:

Ingredients

Canned white beans, drained and rinsed

Fresh spinach leaves

Onion, chopped

Garlic, minced

Low-sodium vegetable broth

Herbs (such as rosemary or sage)

Olive oil

Salt and pepper to taste

Instructions

In a pot, sauté chopped onion and minced garlic until softened.

Add drained white beans and vegetable broth.

Simmer until the beans are heated through.

Stir in fresh spinach leaves and herbs.

Season with salt and pepper.

Serve the spinach and white bean soup.

Mushroom Barley Soup:

Ingredients

Sliced mushrooms

Chopped onion

Carrots, diced

Pearl barley

Low-sodium vegetable broth

Herbs (such as thyme or bay leaf)

Salt and pepper to taste

Instructions

In a pot, sauté chopped onion and sliced mushrooms until browned.

Add diced carrots, pearl barley, and vegetable broth.

Season with herbs, salt, and pepper.

Simmer until barley is tender.

Serve the mushroom barley soup.

Vegetable Noodle Soup:

Ingredients

Assorted vegetables (carrots, celery, onion, etc.), diced

Low-sodium vegetable broth

Noodles of your choice (whole wheat or rice noodles)

Herbs (such as parsley or dill)

Salt and pepper to taste

Instructions

In a pot, sauté diced vegetables until slightly softened.

Add vegetable broth and bring to a simmer.

Add noodles and cook until tender.

Season with herbs, salt, and pepper.

Serve the vegetable noodle soup

Thai Coconut Soup with Tofu and Vegetables:

Ingredients

Tofu, cubed

Assorted vegetables (bell peppers, mushrooms, etc.), sliced

Coconut milk

Low-sodium vegetable broth

Thai red curry paste

Lime juice

Fresh cilantro, chopped

Salt and pepper to taste

Instructions

In a pot, sauté cubed tofu until lightly browned. Set aside.

Sauté sliced vegetables until slightly tender.

Add coconut milk and vegetable broth to the pot.

Stir in Thai red curry paste and simmer.

Return the tofu to the pot and let the flavors meld.

Season with lime juice, chopped cilantro, salt, and pepper.

Serve the Thai coconut soup with tofu and vegetables.

Broccoli and Cheddar Soup:

Ingredients

Broccoli florets

Chopped onion

Vegetable broth

Milk or cream (dairy or plant-based)

Shredded cheddar cheese

Herbs and spices (such as nutmeg or black pepper)

Salt to taste

Instructions

Steam or boil broccoli florets until tender. Set aside.

In a pot, sauté chopped onion until softened.

Add steamed broccoli and vegetable broth.

Use an immersion blender to blend the soup until smooth.

Stir in milk or cream and shredded cheddar cheese.

Season with herbs, spices, and salt.

Heat until cheese is melted and the soup is warmed through.

Serve the broccoli and cheddar soup.

Split Pea Soup with Ham (or Vegetarian Version):

Ingredients

Dried green split peas

Chopped onion

Chopped carrots

Chopped celery

Ham bone or smoked ham (optional, omit for vegetarian version)

Herbs (such as thyme or bay leaf)

Salt and pepper to taste

Instructions

Rinse dried split peas and remove any debris.

In a pot, sauté chopped onion, carrots, and celery until softened.

Add split peas, ham bone or smoked ham (if using), and herbs.

Pour in enough water to cover the ingredients.

Simmer until split peas are tender and the soup thickens.

Remove ham bone, if used, and season with salt and pepper.

Serve the split pea soup.

Roasted Butternut Squash Soup:

Ingredients

Butternut squash, peeled, seeded, and cubed

Chopped onion

Vegetable broth

Herbs and spices (such as cinnamon, nutmeg, or thyme)

Salt and pepper to taste

Olive oil

Instructions

Preheat the oven to 400°F (200°C).

Toss cubed butternut squash with olive oil, herbs, and spices.

Roast squash in the oven until tender and caramelized.

In a pot, sauté chopped onion until softened.

Add roasted butternut squash and vegetable broth.

Blend the soup until smooth using an immersion blender.

Season with salt and pepper.

Serve the roasted butternut squash soup.

Gazpacho with a Sprinkle of Fresh Herbs:

Ingredients

Tomatoes, chopped

Cucumber, peeled and chopped

Red bell pepper, chopped

Red onion, chopped

Garlic, minced

Olive oil

Red wine vinegar

Fresh herbs (such as basil or parsley)

Salt and pepper to taste

Instructions

In a blender, combine chopped tomatoes, cucumber, red bell pepper, red onion, and minced garlic.

Blend until smooth.

While blending, drizzle in olive oil and red wine vinegar.

Season with salt and pepper.

Chill the gazpacho in the refrigerator.

Serve the chilled gazpacho with a sprinkle of fresh herbs.

Potato Leek Soup:

Ingredients

Potatoes, peeled and diced

Leeks, cleaned and sliced

Vegetable broth

Milk or cream (dairy or plant-based)

Herbs (such as thyme or chives)

Salt and pepper to taste

Butter or olive oil

Instructions

In a pot, sauté sliced leeks in butter or olive oil until softened.

Add diced potatoes and vegetable broth.

Simmer until potatoes are tender.

Blend the soup until smooth using an immersion blender.

Stir in milk or cream, herbs, salt, and pepper.

Heat the soup until warmed through.

Serve the potato leek soup.

Cabbage and Sausage Soup:

Ingredients

Sausage links (chicken, turkey, cr plant-based)

Chopped onion

Chopped carrots

Chopped cabbage

Low-sodium chicken or vegetable broth

Herbs (such as thyme or bay leaf)

Salt and pepper to taste

Instructions

In a pot, cook sausage links until browned. Set aside.

Sauté chopped onion, carrots, and cabbage until slightly softened.

Add sliced cooked sausage, broth, and herbs.

Simmer until vegetables are tender and flavors meld.

Season with salt and pepper.

Serve the cabbage and sausage soup.

Corn and Black Bean Chowder:

Ingredients

Corn kernels (fresh, frozen, or canned)

Black beans, drained and rinsed

Chopped onion

Diced potatoes

Vegetable broth

Milk or cream (dairy or plant-based)

Herbs and spices (such as cumin or paprika)

Salt and pepper to taste

Instructions

In a pot, sauté chopped onion until softened.

Add diced potatoes and vegetable broth.

Simmer until potatoes are tender.

Add corn kernels and black beans.

Blend a portion of the soup for creaminess if desired.

Stir in milk or cream, herbs, spices, salt, and pepper.

Heat the chowder until warmed through.

Serve the corn and black bean chowder.

Italian Wedding Soup with Turkey Meatballs:

Ingredients

Ground turkey

Bread crumbs

Chopped onion

Chopped carrots

Chopped spinach

Low-sodium chicken broth

Acini di pepe pasta (or small pasta of your choice)

Fresh parsley, chopped

Parmesan cheese, grated (optional)

Salt and pepper to taste

Instructions

In a bowl, mix ground turkey, bread crumbs, chopped onion, salt, and pepper.

Form the mixture into small meatballs.

In a pot, sauté chopped carrots until slightly softened.

Add low-sodium chicken broth and bring to a simmer.

Add turkey meatballs and acini di pepe pasta.

When meatballs are cooked and pasta is tender, add chopped spinach.

Season with fresh parsley and grated Parmesan cheese if desired.

Serve the Italian wedding soup.

HEMORRHOIDS FRIENDLY DESSERT RECIPES

Fresh Mixed Berries with a Dollop of Yogurt:

Ingredients

Mixed berries (strawberries, blueberries, raspberries, etc.)

Greek yogurt or your choice of yogurt

Instructions

Wash and rinse the mixed berries.

In serving bowls, portion out the mixed berries.

Top each bowl with a dollop of Greek yogurt or your preferred yogurt.

Serve the fresh mixed berries with yogurt.

Baked Apples with Cinnamon and a Drizzle of Honey:

Ingredients

Apples (such as Granny Smith or Honeycrisp)

Ground cinnamon

Honey

Instructions

Preheat the oven to 375°F (190°C).

Core the apples and remove the seeds, leaving the bottom intact.

Sprinkle ground cinnamon inside the apple cavities.

Place the apples in a baking dish and drizzle honey over them.

Bake until the apples are tender, about 25-30 minutes.

Serve the baked apples with a drizzle of honey.

Dark Chocolate Squares with Almonds:

Ingredients

Dark chocolate squares (70% cocoa or higher)

Almonds, whole or chopped

Instructions

Melt the dark chocolate squares using a microwave or double boiler.

While the chocolate is still melted, dip almonds in it or sprinkle them over the melted chocolate.

Place the chocolate-covered almonds on parchment paper to set.

Once the chocolate has hardened, serve the dark chocolate squares with almonds.

Chia Seed Pudding Topped with Fruit:

Ingredients

Chia seeds

Milk (dairy or plant-based)

Sweetener (such as honey, maple syrup, or agave)

Fresh fruit for topping

Instructions

In a bowl, mix chia seeds, milk, and sweetener. Use a ratio of about 1/4 cup chia seeds to 1 cup of milk.

Stir well and let it sit for a few hours or overnight in the refrigerator to thicken.

Once the chia pudding has thickened, portion it into serving dishes.

Top each dish with fresh fruit of your choice.

Serve the chia seed pudding topped with fruit.

Frozen Banana Slices Dipped in Dark Chocolate:

Ingredients

Bananas, sliced

Dark chocolate

Toppings (such as chopped nuts or shredded coconut)

Instructions

Line a baking sheet with parchment paper.

Insert a toothpick into each banana slice and freeze them for a short while.

Melt dark chocolate using a microwave or double boiler.

Dip the frozen banana slices into the melted chocolate, coating them partially.

Sprinkle toppings over the chocolate-coated banana slices.

Place them back on the parchment paper and freeze until the chocolate is set.

Serve the frozen banana slices dipped in dark chocolate.

Greek Yogurt Parfait with Granola and Fruit:

Ingredients

Greek yogurt

Granola

Fresh fruit (berries, sliced banana, etc.)

Honey or maple syrup (optional)

Instructions

In serving glasses or bowls, layer Greek yogurt, granola, and fresh fruit.

Drizzle honey or maple syrup over each layer if desired.

Repeat the layers until the glass or bowl is filled.

Serve the Greek yogurt parfait with granola and fruit.

Rice Pudding Made with Almond Milk and Raisins:

Ingredients

Arborio rice

Almond milk (or any milk of your choice)

Raisins

Sweetener (such as sugar, honey, or agave)

Ground cinnamon

Instructions

In a pot, cook Arborio rice with almond milk over low heat, stirring often.

As the rice cooks and absorbs the milk, add raisins and sweetener to taste.

Continue cooking until the rice is creamy and tender.

Sprinkle ground cinnamon on top before serving.

Serve the rice pudding made with almond milk and raisins.

Fruit Salad with a Squeeze of Citrus:

Ingredients

Assorted fresh fruits (melon, berries, grapes, etc.)

Citrus fruits (orange, grapefruit, lemon, lime)

Fresh mint leaves (optional)

Instructions

Wash, peel, and cut assorted fresh fruits into bite-sized pieces.

In a bowl, combine the mixed fruits.

Squeeze citrus fruits (orange, grapefruit, lemon, lime) over the fruit salad to add a citrusy flavor.

Toss gently to combine.

Garnish with fresh mint leaves if desired.

Serve the fruit salad with a squeeze of citrus.

Baked Pear with a Sprinkle of Cinnamon:

Ingredients

Pears, halved and cored

Ground cinnamon

Honey (optional)

Instructions

Preheat the oven to 375°F (190°C).

Place pear halves, cut-side up, on a baking sheet.

Sprinkle ground cinnamon over the pear halves.

Optionally, drizzle a little honey over each pear half.

Bake until the pears are tender and slightly caramelized, about 20-25 minutes.

Serve the baked pear with a sprinkle of cinnamon.

Oatmeal Cookies with Dried Fruit and Nuts:

Ingredients

Oats

Whole wheat flour

Baking powder

Honey or maple syrup

Dried fruit (raisins, cranberries, etc.)

Chopped nuts (almonds, walnuts, etc.)

Coconut oil or butter

Vanilla extract

Instructions

Preheat the oven to 350°F (175°C).

In a bowl, mix oats, whole wheat flour, and baking powder.

Add honey or maple syrup, dried fruit, chopped nuts, coconut oil or butter, and vanilla extract.

Mix until well combined to form a cookie dough.

Scoop spoonfuls of dough onto a baking sheet and flatten slightly.

Bake until the cookies are golden brown, about 10-12 minutes.

Allow the cookies to cool before serving.

Coconut Milk-Based Ice Cream with Fresh Mango:

Ingredients

Ripe mangoes, peeled and diced

Coconut milk (full-fat)

Sweetener (such as agave or sugar)

Lime juice

Shredded coconut (optional)

Instructions

Blend diced mangoes until smooth.

In a separate bowl, mix coconut milk, sweetener, and lime juice.

Combine the mango puree and coconut milk mixture.

Pour the mixture into an ice cream maker and churn according to the manufacturer's instructions.

Optionally, add shredded coconut during the churning process.

Transfer the ice cream to a container and freeze until firm.

Serve the coconut milk-based ice cream with fresh mango.

Pineapple Sorbet with Mint Leaves:

Ingredients

Pineapple chunks (fresh or frozen)

Sweetener (such as agave or honey)

Fresh mint leaves

Instructions

Blend pineapple chunks until smooth.

Mix in sweetener to taste.

Freeze the pineapple mixture in an ice cream maker according to the manufacturer's instructions.

Scoop the sorbet into serving bowls.

Garnish with fresh mint leaves.

Serve the pineapple sorbet with mint leaves.

Mixed Nut and Dried Fruit Trail Mix:

Ingredients

Assorted mixed nuts (almonds, cashews, etc.)

Dried fruits (apricots, cherries, etc.)

Instructions

Mix together your favorite combination of mixed nuts and dried fruits.

Portion the trail mix into individual servings or a large bowl.

Serve the mixed nut and dried fruit trail mix as a convenient and healthy dessert option.

Baked Peaches with a Hint of Vanilla:

Ingredients

Peaches, halved and pitted

Vanilla extract

Honey (optional)

Cinnamon (optional)

Instructions

Preheat the oven to 375°F (190°C).

Place peach halves, cut-side up, on a baking sheet.

Drizzle a little vanilla extract over each peach half.

Optionally, drizzle honey and sprinkle cinnamon over the peaches.

Bake until the peaches are tender and juicy, about 15-20 minutes.

Serve the baked peaches with a hint of vanilla.

Fresh Watermelon Slices with a Squeeze of Lime:

Ingredients

Watermelon, sliced into wedges

Lime

Instructions

Arrange watermelon slices on a serving platter.

Squeeze fresh lime juice over the watermelon slices.

Serve the fresh watermelon slices with a squeeze of lime.

CHAPTER V: LAST NOTES BEFORE YOU GO!

Our adventure through this hemorrhoids diet cookbook has come to a close, and we'd want to take a moment to thank you for being a part of it. Over the course of these chapters, we've covered the ins and outs of hemorrhoid management via healthy eating habits, delicious recipes, and insightful advice. We hope that the information contained in this cookbook will enable you to better manage your digestive health and alleviate any associated discomfort.

Keep in mind that the process of dealing with hemorrhoids will be different for everyone. Despite the plethora of knowledge and tools supplied by this cookbook, it is still recommended that you see a doctor or dietitian for advice that is particular to your requirements and medical history. Your health is a multifaceted issue, and your healthcare team may offer you assistance that goes far beyond the scope of this cookbook.

Keep in mind that gradual, long-term improvements to your comfort and health may be achieved through a series of tiny, manageable steps. Taking any action toward better health, whether it culinary exploration, nutritional tweaks, or the adoption of more mindful practices, is beneficial.

We don't think anyone should have to make concessions in order to eat in a way that benefits their digestive health and nourishes their body. It has the potential to be a culinary extravaganza, a portal to comfort, and a springboard to permanent happiness. I hope that the knowledge you receive from this cookbook helps you develop a positive and healthy relationship with food and your body.

We appreciate you letting us share in your experience. Comfort, vigor, and the pleasure of enjoying each wholesome bite—may they accompany you throughout your days. Cheers to your well-being and contentment!

The Role of Physical Activity

Beyond its well-known advantages for cardiovascular health and weight control, physical exercise also plays a role in treating hemorrhoids. Maintaining a regular exercise routine is essential for overall digestive health and may help reduce the pain of hemorrhoids.

Constipation is a major cause of hemorrhoid symptoms, but regular physical activity can help relieve the condition and keep bowel motions regular. Hemorrhoids can be prevented or alleviated by engaging in regular physical activity because it increases the muscle contractions of the intestines, which in turn helps transport stool through the digestive tract more effectively.

Hemorrhoid treatment might also benefit from regular exercise to keep a healthy weight. Being overweight might aggravate hemorrhoid pain because it increases pressure on the blood vessels in the anal area. Maintaining or reducing body fat with consistent physical activity and a healthy diet can help ease discomfort and improve quality of life.

Hemorrhoids are only one of many health problems that can result from a sedentary lifestyle, which is linked to poor blood circulation. Regular exercise can help prevent hemorrhoids by increasing blood flow and reducing the irritation and constriction of blood vessels. Physical activity has been shown to improve circulation, which in turn aids recovery and lessens discomfort.

However, it's crucial to remember that not all physical activity is good for people who suffer from hemorrhoids. There should be caution while engaging in activities that require heavy lifting, hard straining, or repetitive trauma to the pelvic region. Walking, swimming, yoga, and stationary cycling are all examples of low-impact workouts that may be easier on the body and less likely to aggravate symptoms.

If you have hemorrhoids or other health issues, you should talk to a doctor before beginning an exercise program or making any changes to an existing one. They may tailor recommendations for workouts, intensity levels, and safety considerations to your specific needs.

You may help your body heal from hemorrhoids and improve your overall health by making exercise a regular part of your routine. Consistency is the key to success in any health pursuit, and by maintaining an active lifestyle, you're making progress toward improved wellbeing.